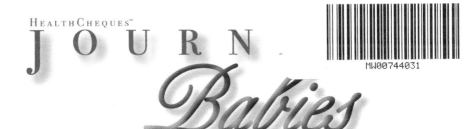

HEALTHCHEQUES™
JOURN
Babies

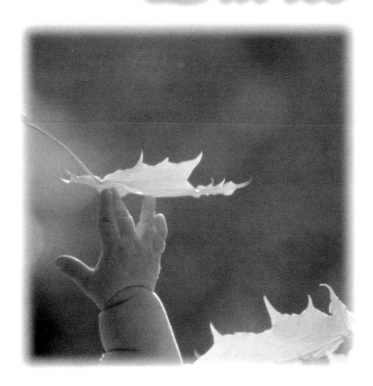

Your Personal Conception & Pregnancy Organizer

MACHELLE SEIBEL, MD
JANE STEPHENSON, RD, CDE
WITH DIANE BADER

Appletree Press, Inc.
151 Good Counsel Drive Suite 125
Mankato, MN 56001
Phone: (507) 345-4848
FAX: (507) 345-3002
Website: www.appletree-press.com

Publisher's Cataloging-in-Publication
(Provided by Quality Books, Inc.)

Seibel, Machelle M.
   HealthCheques, journal babies : your personal
conception & pregnancy organizer / Machelle Seibel, Jane
Stephenson with Diane Bader. -- 1st ed.
   p. cm.
   Includes bibliographical references and index.
   ISBN 1-891011-04-9

   1. Pregnancy--Popular works. 2. Pregnancy--
Miscellanea.   I. Stephenson, Jane. II. Bader, Diane.
III. Title. IV. Title: Journal babies

RG525.S45 2002   618.2
                  QBI102-200565

Appletree Press books are available at special quantity discounts for bulk purchase for sales promotions, premiums, fund-raising,
and educational needs. This book can be customized to meet specific needs. For details—please write, phone, or fax
Appletree Press at the address and contact numbers given at the top of this page.

*The purpose of this book is to educate. While every effort has been made to ensure its accuracy, this book's contents should not be
construed as medical advice. It is sold with the understanding that neither the publisher nor the authors can be held responsible for
any injury caused or alleged to be caused directly or indirectly by the information contained in this book. As each person's health needs
are unique, the reader should consult with his or her physician in all matters relating to health.*

Editors: Diane Bader and Linda Hachfeld
Cover and Book Design: Timothy Halldin, Pike Graphics
Front Cover Photographer: Kenneth Ehlers / ImageState

Printed in the United States of America

Sincere Thanks

To our colleagues, friends, families, and publisher who contributed their time, expertise, and inspiration in the development of HealthCheques™, J o u r n a l.*Babies*: *Your Personal Conception & Pregnancy Organizer.*

We extend a special thanks and acknowledgement to:
Diane Bader for her assistance with the writing, organizing, and editing of the text; *Leigh Bader* for his help creating many of the charts and graphics; *Jackie Boucher*, M.S., R.D., C.D.E., for taking the time out of her busy schedule to help edit and offer expert advice and suggestions; *Linda Hachfeld*, M.P.H., R.D., for her willingness to market and publish yet another HealthCheques™ product; the staff from *Inverness Medical Innovations, Inc.*, for their support and encouragement; *Adrian Seibert* for his assistance with the graphics; *Unipath Diagnostics, Co.*, for providing some of the graphics; *Bridget Swinney*, M.S., R.D., and *Meadowbrook Press* for the rights to use the *Eating Expectantly Food Guide Pyramid*; and *Teresa Novacek* for adding the finishing touches to the final manuscript.

We also wish to thank the following colleagues and friends who generously offered their time to review the text: Janice Abbott; Joan Belluche, B.S., R.N.; Eve Gehling, M.S., R.D., C.D.E.; Wendy Gregor, M.A., R.D., C.D.E.; Elizabeth Haines; Matt Hemingway; Janet Jacobs, F.I.B.S.; Mary McNeil; Stacey Payne, R.D.; Kandi Quarterson; Katie Sheridan; and Kathleen Sheridan.

Machelle Seibel, M.D.
Jane Stephenson, R.D., C.D.E.
Authors

Machelle Seibel, M.D. is a fellow of the American College of Obstetrics and Gynecology and the American Association of Clinical Endocrinologists. He is board certified in obstetrics and gynecology and reproductive endocrinology. Dr. Seibel received his medical degree from the University of Texas, Medical Branch and completed his residency at the Department of Gynecology and Obstetrics at Emory University in Atlanta. He then completed his fellowship in reproductive endocrinology and infertility at Harvard Medical School. Dr. Seibel is a practicing reproductive endocrinologist and medical director of a medical company in the Boston area. Dr. Seibel is also a Professor of Clinical Obstetrics and Gynecology at the University of Massachusetts School of Medicine. He has written, co-authored, and edited more than 200 scientific articles and several books including: *Infertility: Your Questions Answered; Infertility: A Comprehensive Text; Family Building Through Egg and Sperm Donation; Soy: An Alternative to Estrogen for Menopause;* and *A Woman's Book of Yoga.* Dr. Seibel has been voted by a survey of his peers as one of *The Best Doctors in America* in his specialty.

Jane Stephenson, R.D., C.D.E. is a registered dietitian, certified diabetes educator, and nutrition consultant with expertise in women's health issues, cardiovascular disease, weight management, and diabetes. Jane currently works for a medical company in the Boston area. She is author of *HealthCheques™: A Self-Monitoring System* and *Health-Cheques™: A Meal-Planning System.* Jane is co-author of *HealthCheques™: Carbohydrate, Fat & Calorie Guide; Diet-Free HealthCheques™;* and *No-Fuss Diabetes Recipes for 1 or 2.* She was awarded the 2001 *Creative Nutrition Award* for her *HealthCheques™* product line from Diabetes Care and Education (DCE), a practice group of the American Dietetic Association.

CONTENTS

" MAKING THE DECISION

TO HAVE A CHILD —

IT'S MOMENTOUS.

IT IS TO DECIDE FOREVER

TO HAVE YOUR HEART

GO WALKING AROUND

OUTSIDE YOUR BODY. "

Elizabeth Stone

8

JOURNAL BABIES™

Your Personal Conception & Pregnancy Organizer

Name

Address

Phone Hm: Wk:

Health Care Provider's Phone

Date Journal Started

Baby's Due Date

HEALTHCHEQUES™

JOURNAL
Babies

CONCEPTION AND

Pregnancy Guide

INTRODUCTION AND *Welcome*

Welcome to JOURNAL.*Babies*:
Your Personal Conception & Pregnancy Organizer.
There are two parts to this organizer:

Part One: Conception & Pregnancy Guide. This guide will answer many of your questions and concerns about conception and pregnancy. In addition, you will learn about taking care of yourself and your developing baby to ensure the healthiest outcome possible.

Part Two: Conception & Pregnancy Journal. Before conception, use the journal to track the fertile days in your menstrual cycle so you know which days are best for you to try to get pregnant. After conception, record and organize all of the exciting and challenging details surrounding your pregnancy — from conception to delivery. You can also learn about the changes you and your baby are experiencing by reading the month-by-month pregnancy calendar pages.

Bring JOURNAL.*Babies* with you to your doctor's visits as a reference.
After delivery, file it away. Someday you'll want to look back and remember your thoughts, milestones, and pertinent health information related to your pregnancy. You may want to compare pregnancies or share an intimate detail with your partner, a friend, or your child — such as the first time you felt a kick. JOURNAL.*Babies* keeps the memories alive by allowing you to record these details in one convenient place.

How does conception happen?

After sexual intercourse, the sperm begin their journey through the cervix, into the uterus, and out into the fallopian tubes. The sperm and the egg meet in the fallopian tube, where fertilization takes place. For conception to occur, one sperm must penetrate the egg. Several days later, the fertilized egg implants itself into the wall of the uterus.

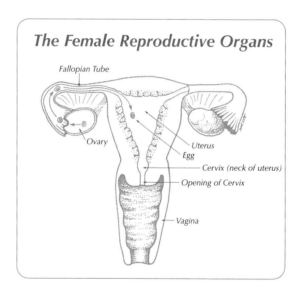

The Female Reproductive Organs

Fallopian Tube

Ovary

Uterus

Egg

Cervix (neck of uterus)

Opening of Cervix

Vagina

When should I stop my birth control if I want to become pregnant?

It's usually recommended that you stop taking birth control pills, stop injections, or have implants removed a few months before you want to become pregnant. It may take several months for your menstrual cycle to become regular. If your cycle was irregular before you began birth control, it may still be irregular after you stop. If you have an intrauterine device (IUD) removed, your physician may recommend waiting until your next cycle to try to conceive.

How do I calculate the number of days in my menstrual cycle?

Your menstrual cycle length is the number of days from the first day of your period to the last day before your next period starts. Cycle day one is the day you get your period. The next day is cycle day two and so on. To calculate your cycle length, start by counting the first day of your menstrual bleeding (not spotting) and stop counting the day before you bleed again on your next cycle. A typical cycle length is 28 days; however, this can vary from month to month and from woman to woman.

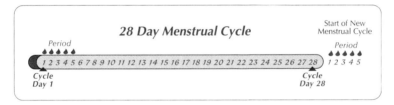

What are the phases of the menstrual cycle?

There are two phases of the menstrual cycle, separated by ovulation. The first phase is called the follicular phase. During this phase, a new egg develops and gets ready for release by your ovary. The days after ovulation are called the luteal phase. The follicular phase can vary, which means the time of ovulation can vary from month to month. The luteal phase remains fairly constant, so once ovulation occurs, your next period will follow in approximately 14 days.

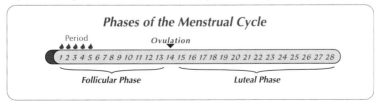

What is meant by a "regular menstrual cycle"?

A regular menstrual cycle generally refers to a cycle that is 26 to 34 days long and occurs about 11 to 13 times per year. Usually the length does not vary by more than four days from one cycle to the next.

What is ovulation?

Ovulation is the process of an egg being released from one of the two ovaries. This generally occurs between the 11th and 17th day of the menstrual cycle. However, this can vary from one woman to another, depending on the length of her menstrual cycles, and can vary in the same woman if her menstrual cycles are irregular.

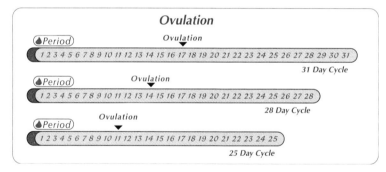

If I have a regular menstrual cycle, does this mean I'm ovulating?

Usually, however, sometimes an egg may only partially develop, and ovulation does not occur.

Can conception occur at any time during my menstrual cycle?

No, there are only a few days during your menstrual cycle when intercourse can lead to pregnancy. Conception is most likely to occur if you have intercourse during ovulation or during the few days leading up to ovulation.

How long does my "fertile period" last?

For most women, the peak fertile period lasts about two to three days. Your egg can only be fertilized for up to 24 hours after ovulation; however, the sperm can live for about 48 to 72 hours. (Sperm have been known to survive for up to five days in sperm-friendly mucus.) Because of this, you have a chance of becoming pregnant from intercourse *before* as well as during ovulation. If your egg is not fertilized, it will be shed during your next menstrual cycle.

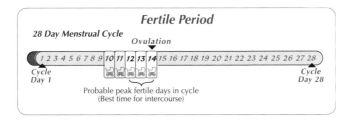

Fertile Period

28 Day Menstrual Cycle

Ovulation

1 2 3 4 5 6 7 8 9 10 11 12 13 14 15 16 17 18 19 20 21 22 23 24 25 26 27 28

Cycle Day 1

Cycle Day 28

Probable peak fertile days in cycle (Best time for intercourse)

Do I release an egg from one ovary one month and the other ovary the next month?

Not necessarily. The chance of either ovary releasing your egg is random, like flipping a coin. In any given cycle, it is impossible to know which ovary will ovulate until about five days before ovulation occurs. At this time, an ultrasound scan will usually show which side the dominant follicle is on.

How can I know if and when I'm ovulating?

There are several ways to find out:

Most reliable
- Use a home ovulation predictor kit to test your urine for a rise in luteinizing hormone (LH) (the hormone that triggers ovulation) or a rise in estrogen, which occurs a few days earlier. Sudden rises in estrogen and LH predict ovulation *before* it occurs.
- Have a blood test done at your physician's office to test for the rise or "surge" in LH.

Less reliable
- Keep a basal body temperature (BBT) chart. Your body temperature rises at least 0.4° Fahrenheit or 1.5° Celsius at the time of ovulation. A BBT shows ovulation *after* it has occurred.

Least reliable
- Track changes in your cervical mucus or saliva. Cervical mucus is generally thick and rubbery before and after ovulation and feels like raw egg whites (thin and slippery) around the time of ovulation. Saliva also undergoes some changes around the time of ovulation. Over-the-counter kits are available for saliva testing, which use a small microscope to look for changes in saliva patterns.
- Experience mid-cycle abdominal pain. Medical studies raise some doubt about this symptom being a true sign of ovulation.
- Have an increase in libido (i.e., sexual desire).

How can a home ovulation predictor test help me if I'm trying to get pregnant?

Knowing when you're going to ovulate helps you time intercourse to increase your chances of getting pregnant. Home ovulation predictor test kits pinpoint the fertile days in your menstrual cycle by testing your urine for a sudden increase in LH (luteinizing hormone) or estrogen and LH, depending on the kit you buy. Ovulation usually occurs within the next three to five days after the rise in estrogen, or within the next one to two days after the rise in LH. This information is very helpful because you then know in advance which days are best to try to get pregnant. (Note: Currently, the only method available for testing estrogen, as well as LH, is the *ClearBlue Easy® Fertility Monitor,* formerly known as *ClearPlan Easy®)*

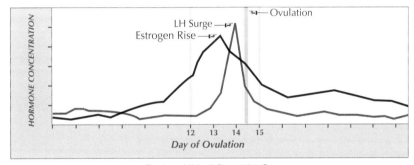

Courtesy of Unipath Diagnostics, Co.

What types of conditions or medications could interfere with the results of my home ovulation predictor test?

If you are actually pregnant, have recently been pregnant, or have reached menopause, you may get a misleading result. The fertility tablet clomiphene citrate (Clomid® or Serophene®) may give a false-positive result with some brands. Therefore, it is often recommended that you wait three days after your last tablet to begin testing. Pain medications, hormone replacement therapy, most antibiotics, antidepressants, street drugs, alcohol, or menstrual bleeding **should not** affect your test results. Check with your doctor if you get unexpected or inconsistent results.

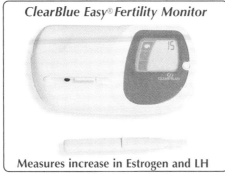

ClearBlue Easy® Fertility Monitor

Measures increase in Estrogen and LH

Courtesy of Unipath Diagnostics, Co.

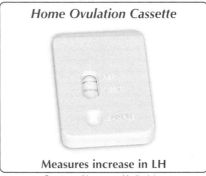

Home Ovulation Cassette

Measures increase in LH

Courtesy of Inverness Medical, Inc.

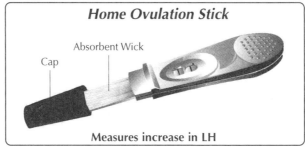

Home Ovulation Stick

Cap

Absorbent Wick

Measures increase in LH

Courtesy of Inverness Medical, Inc.

What is my basal body temperature (BBT), and do I need to buy a special thermometer to take my BBT?

Your BBT is your body's temperature when you first wake up after a good night's sleep. You can buy a special basal thermometer with large, easy-to-read numbers to take your BBT. This usually takes three minutes. However, a digital thermometer may be used instead because it also shows small changes in your body temperature and takes less than one minute.

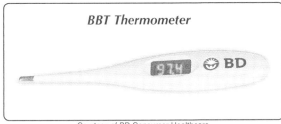

BBT Thermometer

Courtesy of BD Consumer Healthcare

How do I keep a BBT chart, and what does the BBT chart show?

In order to keep a BBT chart, you must measure your temperature each morning, starting with cycle day one of your menstrual cycle (i.e., first day of bleeding). Keep the thermometer by your bed and check your temperature as soon as you wake up, before you get out of bed. You should not eat, drink, or even move around before taking your temperature. Record your temperature every day on a graph or chart (see Monthly Conception Planner, pages 63 to 65) throughout your menstrual cycle. If you plot your BBT for your entire menstrual cycle, you will notice that your temperature usually rises just after ovulation (0.4° Fahrenheit or 1.5° Celsius) and remains this way for the rest of your menstrual cycle. This rise in temperature occurs in response to a rise in the hormone progesterone.

Pictured on the following page are examples of two BBT charts kept by two different women.

- **Graph A** shows a typical ovulation pattern (normal BBT pattern).
- **Graph B** indicates that ovulation did not occur (anovulation BBT pattern).

A) Normal BBT pattern

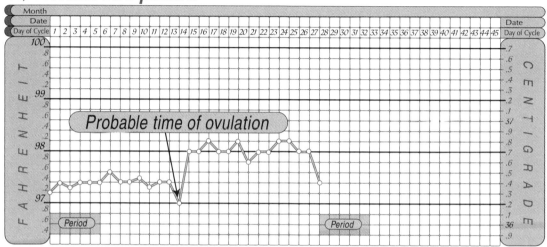

B) Anovulatory BBT pattern

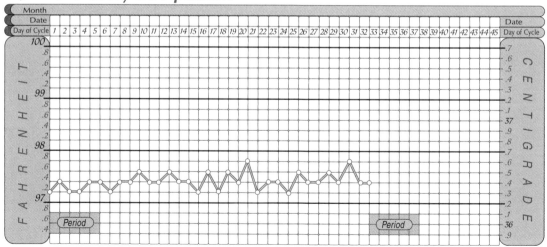

Is charting your BBT a reliable method for timing sexual intercourse?

Probably not. The problem with BBT is that your temperature generally does not rise until ovulation has already occurred. Therefore, you may not have time to plan. It's also important to realize that the BBT rise may be as much as two days off from ovulation. Many couples find it stressful to use BBT for timing sexual intercourse, especially if the temperature pattern rises and falls several times before the actual ovulation rise occurs. BBT is, however, useful in retrospect to see if you had intercourse at the best time or to show ovulation patterns. If your BBT stays elevated for more than 14 days, it suggests that you're pregnant.

What is cervical mucus, and what is its function?

Cervical mucus is a jelly-like substance produced by tiny glands in the cervical canal. It's very responsive to estrogen and progesterone and changes throughout your menstrual cycle and during pregnancy. During most of the menstrual cycle, it's thick like rubber cement and serves as a plug that keeps bacteria out of the uterus. As the middle of the menstrual cycle approaches and the level of estrogen rises in your bloodstream, the cervical mucus becomes more watery and feels like raw egg whites. This allows sperm to live in it like a reservoir and swim through it to get into your uterus. After ovulation, estrogen levels lower and progesterone levels rise, causing the cervical mucus to become thick again.

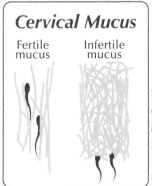

Cervical Mucus

Fertile mucus   Infertile mucus

Illustrated by Pike Graphics

What is spinnbarkeit?

Spinnbarkeit is the term used to describe the stretchiness of cervical mucus. During the middle of the cycle, it may stretch as far as four inches (10 cm). Simply place the mucus between your thumb and first finger and pull your fingers apart. The greater the stretchiness of the mucus, the closer you are to ovulation.

When should I have sexual intercourse in order to increase my chances of getting pregnant?

Having intercourse two to three times around the time of ovulation gives you the best chance of pregnancy. If you're not sure when you ovulate, use an ovulation predictor kit.

If I have intercourse "too often" will it decrease my chances of getting pregnant?

Your chance of pregnancy is reduced only if you have intercourse several times per day because the sperm count decreases. Abstaining from intercourse for a few days may increase the sperm count. However, there is no evidence that this will increase your chances of pregnancy. Abstaining from intercourse for more than five days may actually lower the sperm count.

Does pregnancy always occur if I have intercourse at the right time?

No. The chance of pregnancy in any one cycle is about 15 to 25 percent, even if you and your partner are perfectly fertile and have intercourse at the right time.

Is having an orgasm necessary to get pregnant?

No. You do not need to have an orgasm to conceive.

Is there a particular position during intercourse that is more likely to result in pregnancy?

No. As long as your partner ejaculates into your vagina, the position during intercourse does not have a major impact on your chances of getting pregnant. Contrary to popular belief, elevating your hips and lying still after intercourse does not increase your chances of pregnancy.

Can I time intercourse to increase my chances of having a girl or a boy?

The chances of having a girl or boy is about 50/50. Although experts don't all agree, you may be able to increase the odds to about 60/40 by timing your intercourse. The sperm determines the gender of your child. Every egg carries an X chromosome. Roughly half the sperm also carry an X chromosome, which will result in a girl; while the other half of the sperm carry a Y chromosome, which will result in a boy. Sperm with an X chromosome (girls) swim slower but live longer. Sperm with a Y chromosome (boys) swim faster but don't live as long.

Bottom line: having intercourse closer to ovulation may make it more likely you'll have a boy. To increase the odds of having a girl, have intercourse a few days earlier. (If you want to try this approach, consider using a home ovulation predictor test that measures LH, or estrogen and LH, to time intercourse accordingly.)

Is there a medical procedure available to increase my chances of having a girl or a boy?

Yes, however, it may be expensive. Currently the method of choice for gender selection is preimplantation genetic diagnosis (PGD). PGD involves in vitro fertilization, removing one cell from the developing embryo (which does not hurt the embryo) and testing the chromosomes from that cell to tell the sex of the developing baby. If the embryo is the desired gender, it's transferred into the woman's uterus. These methods are extremely accurate. Another method of gender selection is the separation of the X and Y chromosomes from sperm. Separation methods, though much less costly than PGD, are still expensive and have a success rate of approximately 75 to 90 percent. Gender selection procedures have been a source of controversy for years due to the ethical, moral, and legal issues surrounding them.

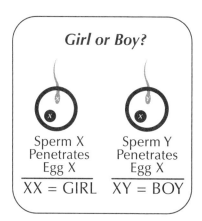

How many sperm must be ejaculated for pregnancy to occur?

No one knows for sure. In theory, only one is needed. However, a low sperm count or poor quality sperm may make it more difficult for you to become pregnant. In general, the lower the sperm count, the longer it takes for pregnancy to occur.

How and why does my partner collect a semen sample?

There are two ways: either by masturbation into a clean container or by having intercourse using special sperm collection condoms. Either way, the sample should be kept at body temperature and brought in before one hour if it's not collected in a doctor's office. The semen sample gives a good idea of your partner's level of fertility.

How many sperm are released during intercourse?

On average, 100 to 300 million are deposited in the vagina at the time of ejaculation. Sperm counts are usually described as number of millions of sperm per milliliter of fluid (five milliliters equals one teaspoon). The volume of the usual ejaculate is three to five milliliters.

Why are so many sperm released if only one is needed to fertilize the egg?

Many sperm are lost along the way. Fewer than 25 actually reach the egg and usually only one succeeds in fusing with the egg.

It seems like most of the sperm leak out after intercourse. Is this a problem?

No. After intercourse, some of the sperm remain within the vagina, stuck in the mucus of the cervix. Sperm living in the cervical mucus will not fall out.

I've had my tubes tied (tubal ligation), but now I want to have a baby. Is this possible?

Yes. Tubes can be surgically repaired (tubal reanastamosis). Depending on the type of tubal ligation you had, when it was done, your partner's sperm count, your age, and the skill of your surgeon, success rates may reach more than 80 percent. You can also become pregnant with in vitro fertilization if surgery isn't successful or if you want to avoid surgery.

My partner has had a vasectomy, and now we want to have a child. Is this possible?

Yes, it may be possible if he has the vasectomy reversed. Depending on the type of vasectomy he's had, when it was done, his sperm count, and the skill of his surgeon, success rates may be as high as 80 percent. You can also become pregnant with in vitro fertilization if surgery isn't successful. This does require your partner to undergo a minor operation to remove his sperm from the testicle.

What else must I do to prepare myself for getting pregnant?

Focus on health: Preparing for pregnancy is a great time to focus on good nutrition, a healthy active lifestyle, weight management, and stress management. It's also important to begin taking a folic acid supplement at least three months before trying to conceive. This vitamin can help prevent neural tube birth defects such as spina bifida. Stop smoking and/or taking street drugs at least six months before trying to become pregnant. It's also best to eliminate or cut down on alcohol and caffeine.

See your doctor: Get a checkup with your primary care doctor, gynecologist, or midwife. This is a good time to make sure your Pap smear and vaccines (e.g., German measles/rubella) are up to date and to discuss any other health concerns. If you're taking any prescription or over-the-counter medications, herbal remedies, and/or dietary supplements, ask your doctor if it's dangerous to take them during conception and/or pregnancy.

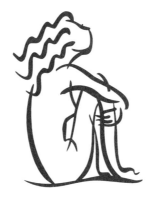

What are some of the reasons that I may not be getting pregnant?

You may not be giving yourself enough time. Eighty-five percent of couples will conceive after one year of unprotected intercourse. If you're older, it might take longer. If you're using a lubricant, be certain it doesn't kill sperm. Also, be sure you're having intercourse during your fertile time. If you haven't gotten pregnant within one year of trying, it's time for you and your partner to see your doctor. Older women are encouraged to see their physician after six months of fertility focused intercourse, as time is not on their side. See your doctor right away if you have a medical condition or suspect a problem (e.g., if you're not getting periods or if you have irregular periods).

What is infertility?

Infertility can be defined as the inability to get pregnant after one year of unprotected intercourse. Of course, some couples will take longer than one year but will eventually get pregnant without a doctor's help.

- *For men,* infertility can stem from a low sperm count, no sperm count, abnormal sperm, or sperm with reduced motility. Sometimes sexual difficulties, such as premature ejaculation or impotence, can also be the problem.

- *For women,* difficulties may arise when anti-sperm antibodies are found in cervical mucus, making it extremely difficult for sperm to survive. Some women may not be ovulating or ovulate infrequently. Endometriosis, a blockage or scarring of the fallopian tubes, polycystic ovary syndrome, or abnormalities in the uterus, such as fibroids, can also contribute to infertility in women.

Are there national support groups for infertility?

Organizations such as the *American Infertility Association* and *RESOLVE* are national organizations with local chapters to assist women and men with infertility issues.

The American Infertility Association
Toll-free phone: (888) 917-3777
www.americaninfertility.com

RESOLVE: The National Infertility Assoc.
Toll-free phone: (888) 623-0744
www.resolve.org

What is endometriosis? Can this cause infertility?

The lining of the uterus is called the endometrium. When it sheds into the vagina each month, some of the uterine lining cells may flow backwards through the fallopian tubes into the pelvis and stick to the pelvic organs. This is called endometriosis. Like transplanted grass, the abnormally placed uterine lining grows and menstruates each month. This can cause scarring, painful menstrual periods, painful intercourse, and reduced fertility. Sometimes cysts of endometriosis called endometriomas grow inside the ovaries. If your doctor suspects endometriosis, a laparoscopy (day surgery using a telescope through a small belly button incision) is required to make the diagnosis. Treatment can usually be done at the same time. Several medications are also available to treat endometriosis by preventing menstruation and shrinking the abnormal tissues.

Do women become less fertile as they grow older?

Yes, getting pregnant takes a little longer with increasing age. For instance, it takes a woman 25 years of age or younger, on average, two to three months to get pregnant, compared with six months or more for a woman who is 35 years of age or older. For men, the decline in fertility is small and generally occurs after the age of 60.

Can I get pregnant if I have only one healthy tube?

Yes, it's still possible to conceive if you have only one healthy tube; however, it may take longer.

What is clomiphene and how does it work?

Clomiphene citrate (Clomid® or Serophene®) is a drug used to stimulate the ovaries to ovulate. One or more tablets are generally given within the first five days of the menstrual cycle, and a course of treatment usually lasts for five days.

How can gonadotropins help me to conceive?

Gonadotropin means literally "stimulate the gonads." The two gonadotropins, follicle-stimulating hormone (FSH) and LH are injections that promote egg growth and development in women and sperm development in men. Gonadotropins are usually given for six to ten days in the first half of a woman's menstrual cycle or two to three times per week for men. Some of these drugs include: Gonal-F®, Fertinex®, Follistim®, Pergonal®, Humegon®, and Repronex®.

When should I start to think about assisted conception as an option?

If you've been trying to get pregnant for several years and haven't been successful, if fertility testing has revealed that it's unlikely you'll be able to become pregnant on your own, or if you're trying to get pregnant without a partner, assisted conception may be an option. These procedures can be expensive and may or may not be covered under various insurance plans.

I'm ready to try assisted conception. What are my options?

Intrauterine Insemination (IUI): An IUI is often done when the man has an abnormal sperm count, the woman does not make enough cervical mucus, or the couple has unexplained infertility. Gonadotropin hormones are given to the woman during the first half of the menstrual cycle to increase the number of developing eggs. As the eggs approach maturity, an injection of human chorionic gonadotropin (hCG) pregnancy hormone is given. Sperm is then collected, washed in the laboratory, placed into a catheter, and passed through the cervix into the uterus.

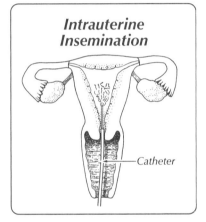

Intrauterine Insemination

Catheter

In Vitro Fertilization (IVF): IVF is commonly referred to as the "test-tube baby" treatment and is generally used when tubes are blocked or badly damaged, but it can also be used for other reasons. Gonadotropin hormones are given to the woman during the first half of the menstrual cycle to increase the number of developing eggs. As the eggs approach maturity, an injection of hCG is given before the eggs are collected to help them mature and to time their collection. Eggs are removed with the help of an ultrasound using local anesthesia and are then fertilized by sperm in the laboratory. Two or three fertilized eggs are then transferred back into the uterus through the cervix.

Gamete Intra-Fallopian Transfer (GIFT): The main difference between IVF and GIFT is that fertilization takes place in the fallopian tubes instead of in the laboratory. Therefore, you must have at least one open tube to be a candidate for GIFT. Your eggs (or donor eggs) and sperm are placed into a catheter outside of the body and then injected back into the fallopian tube. The first few steps are similar to IVF, including stimulating the ovaries with drugs, monitoring follicle growth, giving an hCG injection, and collecting the eggs.

Intra Cytoplasmic Sperm Injection (ICSI): ICSI is used as a part of IVF. It helps fertilization occur by injecting a single sperm directly into an egg's cytoplasm (i.e., the white of an egg). This requires doing in vitro fertilization first to gather the eggs. After ICSI, the fertilized eggs are transferred back into the uterus.

Assisted Hatching: After fertilization, the eggshell must open (hatch) so that the fertilized egg can burrow into the uterine lining and implant. If the eggshell is too thick, or a woman is in her later reproductive years, a scientist may make an opening in the fertilized eggshell after in vitro fertilization, to assist the hatching process.

Blastocyst Transfer: Fertilized eggs that develop to the blastocyst stage are more likely to lead to a pregnancy than fertilized eggs that stop developing. After fertilization, the fertilized egg is called an embryo for the first three days or so. With time, the number of cells increase, and the embryo forms a fluid filled center. This stage is called a blastocyst. Many IVF centers now allow fertilized eggs to grow more than three days so they can choose only the blastocyst stage embryos for transfer. Usually only two are transferred to prevent more than twins from being born.

How successful is assisted conception?

The success rates range from 15 to 35 percent, depending on the cause of your infertility, your age, and the treatment you receive. After age 40, success rates are lower.

I think I might be pregnant. How can I find out?

There are three ways to find out if you're pregnant: urine test, blood test, or ultrasound. The most popular method is a urine test. This can be done at home using a pregnancy test kit, and the results are immediate. A blood test can be done in your doctor's office; sometimes the results take a few days. Although not as common, an ultrasound can also be used when you are at least one to two weeks late on your menstrual period. This will not only confirm your pregnancy, but also help determine your due date.

How does a home pregnancy test work?

Home pregnancy test kits are designed to detect the pregnancy hormone called hCG in your urine. HCG is a hormone that is produced by the placenta of the developing fetus.

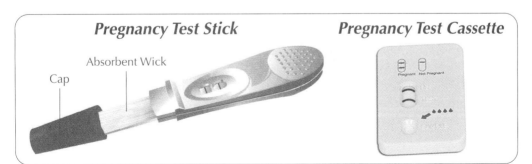

Courtesy of Inverness Medical, Inc.

How soon can I take a home pregnancy test?

A home pregnancy test *may* be positive three to four days before your period is due, but this is often too early to test. To be certain that the pregnancy hormone (hCG) can be detected in your urine, most home pregnancy tests advise you to test the day after your missed period (approximately two weeks after conception). If you test too early and you get a negative result, wait a few days and re-test.

I'm late for my period, but my home pregnancy test is negative. What should I do?

First, double check to see that you are not testing too early after conception, that the test hasn't expired, and that you followed the instructions properly. Also, excessive fluid intake could dilute the hCG in your urine, causing a false-negative test result. Wait a few days and then test again. You may want to re-test with your first morning urine because it's the most concentrated. If you still do not get your period, consult your physician. Other than pregnancy, your period may be late for a variety of reasons, such as, stress, excessive exercise, significant changes in your body weight, and/or a hormonal imbalance.

What types of conditions or medications could interfere with the results of my home pregnancy test?

If you recently gave birth, miscarried, terminated a pregnancy, or are taking hCG pregnancy hormone injections (e.g., APL®, Pregnyl®, Profasi®), you may show a false-positive test result. Also, certain health conditions, such as ovarian cysts, may cause a false result. Birth control pills, painkillers, antibiotics, hormone replacement therapy, antidepressants, street drugs, alcohol, breastfeeding, or menstrual bleeding ***should not*** affect your test results. Check with your doctor if you get unexpected or inconsistent results.

How soon can I take a blood pregnancy test?

Blood pregnancy tests are often accurate as early as seven to ten days after conception. These tests are performed at your doctor's office or clinic.

Is it possible to get periods while I'm pregnant?

Some women have "period-like" bleeding during their pregnancy, especially early pregnancy. However, you should check with your doctor if you experience any bleeding during your pregnancy because it could suggest that there is a problem with the pregnancy.

What are some of the early signs of pregnancy?

Early Signs of Pregnancy	
Missed menstrual period	Fatigue
Upset stomach or bloating	Sensitivity to tastes and smells
Light menstrual period or spotting	Nausea or morning sickness
Feeling emotional	Food cravings
Tender or swollen breasts	Frequent urination
Constipation	Metallic taste in mouth

How much weight should I gain during my pregnancy?

Recommended Weight Gain During Pregnancy
If you're average weight: 25 to 35 pounds
If you're underweight: 28 to 40 pounds
If you're overweight: 15 to 25 pounds
If you're carrying twins: 35 to 45 pounds

Recommended Pattern of Weight Gain During Pregnancy
First trimester: 2 to 4 pounds
Second trimester: About 1 pound per week
Third trimester: About 1 pound per week

Where does all the weight go?

Approximately one-third of your weight gain is the fetus, placenta (afterbirth), and amniotic fluid (the liquid surrounding your baby). Your enlarged breasts, womb, extra body fat, and increased blood and fluids account for the rest. Here are some average numbers:

Where the Weight Goes	
Baby	7 1/2 pounds
Womb (uterus)	2 pounds
Breasts	2 pounds
Placenta	1 1/2 pounds
Fat	4 to 14 pounds
Amniotic fluid	2 pounds
Increased blood & fluid	6 to 8 pounds

How will I know when my baby is due?

Pregnancy usually lasts 40 weeks from your last menstrual period. A simple way to calculate the approximate due date is to subtract three months from the date of your last menstrual period and add seven days to that date. For example, if your last period was April 15 (first day of menstrual bleeding), your baby should be due about January 22. Only about one in 20 babies are born on their due date.

How often will I see my doctor during my pregnancy?

Your doctor will probably see you for your first visit between your sixth and eighth week of pregnancy. You will then be seen monthly until 28 weeks, every other week until 36 weeks, and once a week until you deliver.

What kinds of routine tests will I have during my pregnancy?

During each of your prenatal visits, your weight and blood pressure will be recorded. You will be asked to provide a urine specimen, which will be checked for protein, glucose (blood sugar), and ketones (substances found in your urine when you haven't eaten enough or have uncontrolled diabetes). Periodic blood tests will be done to rule out other conditions, such as gestational diabetes (a type of diabetes mothers may develop during pregnancy).

My doctor has diagnosed me with gestational diabetes. What does this mean?

Gestational diabetes is a type of diabetes that occurs only during pregnancy. It does increase your chances of developing diabetes later on. Gestational diabetes happens when your body does not make enough insulin to control your blood glucose (sugar) level. When you eat a meal, your body breaks down the food you eat into a simple sugar called "glucose". If you don't have enough insulin to carry the glucose into your cells for energy, the excess glucose stays in your bloodstream and your blood glucose level gets too high. The excess blood glucose can cross the placenta and cause harm to your developing baby.

To manage your blood glucose level, you will need to follow a meal plan to help control the amount of carbohydrate you eat and drink. Carbohydrates can be found in many foods, such as, milk, fruits, vegetables, breads, cereals, candy, potatoes, rice, and pasta. If your blood glucose level cannot be controlled with diet alone, you may need to take insulin injections. A certified diabetes educator (C.D.E.) or registered dietitian (R.D.) can help design a meal plan for you. To locate an R.D. in your area, contact The American Dietetic Association's referral service by calling 1-800-366-1655 or visit the website at www.eatright.org.

Why is my blood type checked during my pregnancy?

It's important to identify your blood type for two reasons: in case you need a blood transfusion and to check your Rhesus, or "Rh" factor to see if your blood is Rh positive or Rh negative. If you are Rh negative and the father of your child is Rh positive, problems can arise if your baby is Rh positive, as well. Your body might react to your baby's Rh positive blood by making antibodies — as if it were allergic to it. These antibodies can cross the placenta and harm the fetus. This is generally not a problem with your first pregnancy because it takes time for the antibodies to build up in your blood. Your doctor will give you an Rh immune globulin (RhIg) injection right after birth to help prevent Rh problems with future pregnancies. The injection may also be given during your pregnancy.

What else can I expect at my prenatal visits?

At your first visit, you can expect to have a physical exam, including a pelvic exam, and a complete health history. At this time and at all future visits, your abdomen (belly) will be measured to check the height of the womb (fundus) and the growth of the fetus. Your baby's heartbeat will be routinely checked after your 12th week of pregnancy.

What kinds of special tests are available if I need them?

If you're at risk, or have a family history of certain diseases such as, diabetes, AIDS, sickle cell anemia, thalassemia (a blood disorder that causes anemia), or toxoplasmosis (an infection caused by a parasite found in contaminated cat and animal feces), your doctor may order special blood tests. There are also tests available that may indicate possible problems with the fetus. (See chart on next page.)

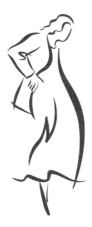

Special Tests Available

Name of Test	Type of Test	When Test is Done
Maternal serum screening AFP test	Blood test for screening neural tube defects (spina bifida) or Down's syndrome.	15 to 18 weeks
Ultrasound	Imaging of fetus from sound waves. Gives information about the fetus such as, age, growth, placenta placement, fetal position, movement, heart rate, number of fetuses, and may detect some problems.	Any time throughout the pregnancy
Amniocentesis	A sample of amniotic fluid is taken from the womb through the abdomen with a fine needle and tested for genetic and chromosomal problems. It also can reveal the sex of the baby and lung maturity.	15 to 18 weeks (May be recommended for women over the age of 35)
Chorionic villus sampling (CVS)	Similar to amniocentesis, except a small piece of the placenta is removed with a needle through the cervix. It also tests for genetic and chromosomal problems, but the test can be done earlier in the pregnancy.	10 to 12 weeks

What is "crown to rump" length and why is it used to describe the length of my baby during pregnancy?

The length of the embryo from its head to its tail is called the crown to rump length. During the early weeks of pregnancy, the embryo is quite small and curled up. In the first 12 weeks, all embryos grow at the same pace. By measuring the embryo's length from crown to rump, the approximate number of weeks of the fetus can be determined. As your baby develops, his or her legs form and are tucked up in the fetal position. The length is still measured crown to rump, or head to baby's bottom. Once your baby is born, he or she will be measured from head to toe.

Is it safe to have sex while I'm pregnant?

Sexual intercourse is not harmful to your baby. Your baby is protected by a cushion of amniotic fluid. This fluid-filled sac is deep within your womb. Therefore, even deep penile penetration is safe. Toward the end of your pregnancy, intercourse may become quite cumbersome, so try to find positions that are comfortable for your changing body. Although sex is usually safe for most couples, your doctor may advise you to abstain from sexual intercourse if you have a history of miscarriage, unexplained bleeding, placenta previa (when the placenta or "afterbirth" covers the cervix), or premature labor.

What kinds of foods should I be eating during my pregnancy?

When it comes to eating healthy during your pregnancy, use The *Eating Expectantly Food Guide Pyramid* (pictured below) to help you build a healthy diet. Try to choose the recommended number of servings from each of the five food groups so you don't miss out on any key nutrients, such as, calcium, protein, fiber, or iron. Include nutrient-rich foods in your diet daily such as whole grains, fresh fruits, vegetables, lean meats, and dairy products. Eat fats and sweets in moderation.

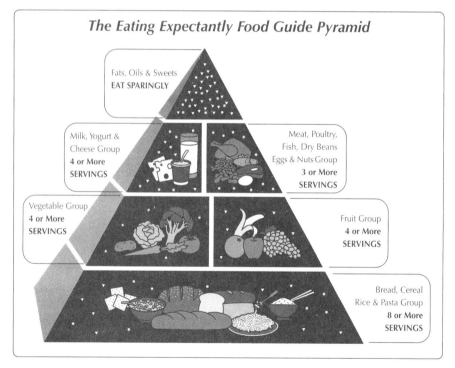

The Eating Expectantly Food Guide Pyramid

Fats, Oils & Sweets
EAT SPARINGLY

Milk, Yogurt & Cheese Group
4 or More SERVINGS

Meat, Poultry, Fish, Dry Beans Eggs & Nuts Group
3 or More SERVINGS

Vegetable Group
4 or More SERVINGS

Fruit Group
4 or More SERVINGS

Bread, Cereal Rice & Pasta Group
8 or More SERVINGS

Source: Modified for pregnancy based on the Food Guide Pyramid from the U.S. Department of Agriculture/U.S. Department of Health and Human Services. From *Eating Expectantly: A Practical and Tasty Guide to Prenatal Nutrition* by Bridget Swinney, M.S., R.D., Meadowbrook Press, 2000. www.Healthyfoodzone.com.

What if I don't like to drink milk or eat dairy products? Are there other sources of calcium?

During pregnancy, calcium lowers the risk of high blood pressure, leg cramps, and pre-term birth. Both you and your baby need calcium for healthy bones and teeth. Thus, if you don't eat enough foods containing calcium, your body will take calcium from your bones to meet the needs of your baby — putting your bones and teeth at risk. You can eat other calcium-rich foods, such as, broccoli, greens (e.g., spinach, kale, collard greens), calcium-fortified juices, calcium-fortified soy products, and salmon with bones.

However, if you don't eat at least three servings of calcium-rich foods each day, consider taking a calcium supplement, but keep in mind your body generally absorbs calcium from foods better. Supplements containing calcium phosphate, calcium citrate, or calcium carbonate are absorbed the best. If you decide to take a calcium supplement, take it separately (one to two hours apart) from your prenatal vitamin because calcium interferes with the absorption of iron in your prenatal vitamin.

What if I'm lactose intolerant and can't tolerate milk or dairy products?

If you have trouble digesting the milk sugar called lactose — don't give up on milk and dairy products. The good news is you may be able to tolerate more lactose during your pregnancy. Try cheese, yogurt with active cultures, buttermilk, and sweet acidophilus milk. The enzyme "lactase" which breaks down milk sugar is also available in over-the-counter drops (to add to milk) or pills (to take before eating dairy or drinking milk). You can also purchase lactase-treated milk.

How many extra calories do I need to eat now that I'm pregnant?

During your first trimester, you don't need to eat any extra calories. During your second and third trimesters, your body only needs an extra 300 calories each day for your baby's growth and development. This is roughly equivalent to an average-sized sandwich or one slice of cheese pizza. You're not really eating for two, so watch those extra calories if you want to avoid excess weight gain.

Can I drink beverages with caffeine during my pregnancy?

There's not enough information about the amount of caffeine that is safe to consume during pregnancy. To be safe, limit caffeinated beverages — such as, coffee, tea, and caffeinated soda — to two cups per day or fewer. Caffeine acts as a stimulant and may cause blood vessels to tighten and the heart rates of you and your baby to increase. It also has a mild diuretic effect, causing fluid loss. Caffeine is found in some beverages, foods, and medications. Decaffeinated beverages, milk, water, and juice are other options.

Can I drink diet soft drinks during my pregnancy?

Aspartame (NutraSweet®), the sweetener found in many soft drinks, has not been shown to cause birth defects, so experts consider moderate use — one to two servings per day or fewer — safe during pregnancy.

Are there any foods I should avoid or limit during my pregnancy?

Avoid raw and undercooked meats and fish and unpasteurized dairy products. To ensure that you destroy any unwanted bacteria — such as salmonella, toxoplasmosis, and e-coli — cook meats, fish, poultry, and eggs thoroughly. Some research shows that it may be best to limit or avoid swordfish, shark, and tuna due to high levels of mercury found in these fish. You should also limit liver and liver pâté because the high level of vitamin A found in these foods could be toxic to the fetus.

What other kinds of things can harm my developing baby?

There are several things you should avoid during pregnancy to ensure the best possible outcome for your baby. Listed below are some of the most common "don'ts" during pregnancy.

Think before you drink: Alcohol crosses the placenta and enters your baby's blood stream. Excessive alcohol consumption may cause serious birth defects. As little as one drink a day has been shown to decrease birth weight. To be on the safe side, avoid alcohol entirely during your pregnancy.

Stop smoking: Did you know that babies born to smoking moms weigh an average of one-half pound less than babies born to non-smoking moms? It's true. Kick the habit for the health of your baby and yourself. In addition to causing lower birth weight, smoking reduces the amount of oxygen and nutrients that cross the placenta to your baby and increases the risk of premature birth and miscarriage. If you need help quitting, talk to your health care provider about your options.

Beware of cat and pet litter: The parasite that causes the infection toxoplasmosis can be found in some animal feces (such as cat feces), and some raw or undercooked meats. Toxoplasmosis can cause blindness, mental retardation, and deafness to your unborn child if you are infected during your pregnancy. Playing with the cat is not a problem. However, have someone else clean the litter box. Also, if you like to garden, dirt can be contaminated with feces; so wear garden gloves.

Say no to drugs: All drugs, illegal or legal, can potentially be harmful to your baby. Consult your health care provider before taking any medication, herbal remedy, or dietary supplement. Even an aspirin or an over-the-counter cold remedy should be pre-approved.

Avoid x-rays during pregnancy: It's possible that x-rays could harm your baby, especially during the first trimester. If you're scheduled for any x-rays, such as routine dental x-rays, hold off until after delivery, if possible, or be sure to wear a lead apron.

Morning sickness is making it difficult for me to eat healthy. Do you have any suggestions?

If you experience morning sickness during your pregnancy, the good news is that it usually disappears or subsides by the second trimester. However, some women have morning sickness on and off during their entire pregnancy. Despite its name, morning sickness can occur at any time of the day or night. The nausea and/or vomiting associated with morning sickness can make eating and drinking a challenge. Before you try alternative remedies or medications for morning sickness, check with your health care provider. Listed on the next page are some tips for morning sickness survival.

Drink plenty of fluids: Dehydration from not drinking enough fluids and/or vomiting can be one of the most serious concerns of morning sickness. Try to drink at least eight to 10 cups of fluid each day. It may be helpful to drink fluids between meals rather than with meals. Popsicles, sparkling water, ginger ale, lemonade, soda, and fruit smoothies may be more easily tolerated.

Eat small, frequent meals with snacks in between: Try some dry carbohydrate foods such as, crackers or cereal before you get out of bed to help reduce nausea and vomiting. Eat small frequent meals throughout the day and drink fluids between meals to help keep food down. It may help to avoid greasy, spicy, and strong smelling foods.

Eat what you can, when you can: Use common sense when it comes to managing your morning sickness. Find out what kinds of foods you can and can't tolerate during different times of the day. If you find yourself reaching for something not-so-nutritious to curb your nausea, don't feel guilty, sometimes it's more important to "just keep something down". Take advantage of the times when you can eat healthier foods and stock up! If you can't handle the sight, smell, or taste of meat, try some meatless alternatives, such as soy cheese, soy yogurt, or a vegetarian burger to boost your protein intake. Continue to take your prenatal vitamin. If you can't handle it first thing in the morning or on an empty stomach, take it during the day with food, or before bedtime.

I seem to be urinating more frequently. Should I cut back on drinking fluids?
No. You need to stay well hydrated during your pregnancy. If you find yourself making several trips to the bathroom in the middle of the night, cut back on fluids in the evening hours. Sleeping on your side may also help to relieve some of the pressure on your bladder.

I've been constipated during my pregnancy. What can I do about this?

Constipation is a common problem caused by pregnancy hormones and compounded by the amount of iron in some prenatal vitamins. To help control constipation, eat plenty of high fiber foods, such as whole grain cereals, fruits, and vegetables; drink plenty of fluid; and stay physically active.

My feet and ankles have been swelling, especially at the end of the day. What can I do about this?

Mild swelling in your feet and ankles is very common during your second and third trimesters. Notify your doctor if the swelling is severe, doesn't go away within a 24 hour period, if the swelling is also present in your face and/or hands, or is accompanied by sudden weight gain.

Here Are a Few Tips to Keep the Swelling Under Control

- Continue to drink plenty of fluid.
- Avoid long periods of standing.
- Elevate your feet while sitting.
- Sleep on your left side.
- Limit your salt intake.
- Wear pregnancy support hose and avoid elastic-top stockings or socks.

Can I exercise during my pregnancy?

Yes, regular exercise is beneficial and should be done with your doctor's approval. Gentle exercises done on a regular basis, such as walking, swimming, and yoga may help you become more fit, be more mentally alert, sleep better, and feel better about yourself in general. Exercise videos designed for pregnant women can be a great way to stay active in the privacy of your home. Prenatal exercise classes are also available at many fitness clubs. If you are already an avid exerciser, you should continue with your typical workout routine unless you are participating in a dangerous or very strenuous sport (e.g., downhill skiing, sprinting, or ironman marathons). If you have never exercised before, you should start slowly and build up gradually to increase your stamina.

Guidelines For Exercising Safely During Pregnancy

- Exercise with a friend when possible.
- Warm up and cool down properly (including stretching).
- Drink plenty of fluids before, during, and after exercise.
- Monitor your heart rate.
- Dress for the weather and avoid exercising in the heat.
- Wear proper footwear.
- Listen to your body when it needs to rest.
- Stop exercising immediately and consult your doctor if you have pain, vaginal bleeding, feel unusually faint, dizzy, or short of breath.

What circumstances could prevent me from exercising?

Your doctor may recommend that you avoid vigorous exercise entirely with some medical conditions: carrying multiple births, cardiac disease, placenta previa (when the placenta or "afterbirth" covers the cervix), ruptured membranes, incompetent cervix, premature labor, or history of miscarriages. Some medical conditions that may limit your physical activities are: high blood pressure diabetes, history of bleeding, history of premature labor, or cardiac arrhythmia. Again, talk to your health care provider before starting an exercise program.

What is the fluid leaking from my breasts?

A watery fluid called "colostrum" may leak from your breasts, particularly in the third trimester. This is the first milk your body produces in preparation for breastfeeding. It contains vitamins, minerals, and protective antibodies for your baby. Not every woman will leak colostrum before delivery.

How do twins develop?

Twins develop very early in pregnancy, shortly after the sperm and egg unite. About 80 percent of twins are fraternal. This happens when two separate sperm fertilize two separate eggs at the same time. These embryos develop with separate placentas. Fraternal twins may look very different and be different sexes.

Identical twins occur when one egg is fertilized by one sperm and then splits into two embryos. Identical twins have only one placenta, are always the same sex, and contain the same genetic material.

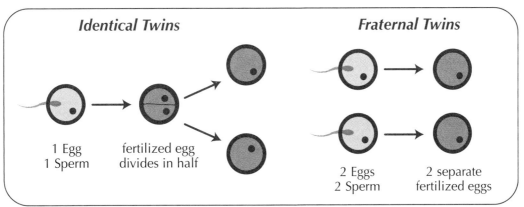

Illustrated by Pike Graphics

What kinds of things should I think about as I prepare for labor and delivery?
You may want to develop your own personal childbirth plan and discuss it with your doctor or midwife. On page 99, you can record your childbirth plan in detail. Listed below are some typical things to think about before you deliver your baby. Keep in mind that some of the items may not apply to you or may not be a choice, depending on hospital policy.

Things to Think About for Labor and Delivery
Will you attend childbirth education classes?
Will you deliver at home, in a hospital, or birthing center?
Who will drive you to the hospital?
Who will be your childbirth partner and coach?
Will anyone else be present at your birth (e.g., siblings, friends, relatives)?
Will you allow medical students to be present?
What position would you prefer for delivery?
Have you learned various breathing techniques to use during labor and delivery?
Would you like to be offered medication for pain relief, such as, an epidural (anesthesia that numbs your abdomen); or a narcotic drug injection, such as, meperidine (Demerol®)?
Who will cut the umbilical cord?
Would you like to have your baby placed directly on your abdomen immediately following delivery?
Would you prefer an episiotomy (a cut made to the perineum to make room for the baby to be born vaginally) or do you want to take the risk of tearing naturally?
Will you allow a camcorder or camera in the delivery room?
Would you like to watch your baby being delivered?
Do you want your baby to stay in the room with you (birth in) if hospital policy allows?
Will you breastfeed, bottle feed, or a combination of the two?
If you have a boy, will you have him circumcised?

How can I tell if labor has begun?

Labor is under way when your uterus starts to contract regularly, causing your cervix (opening of your womb) to dilate. If your contractions are only once or twice per hour, wait a while; true labor has not begun. Once contractions become regular and less than 30 minutes apart, call your doctor or midwife.

How do I know if I'm in false labor?

False labor contractions are generally referred to as "Braxton-Hicks' contractions". These practice contractions help prepare your uterus to go into true labor. They can occur as early as the second trimester and can be quite regular, although they're usually irregular and fade away after an hour or two. True labor usually begins slowly and builds into regular contractions that are more painful and come closer together.

What is a "bloody show"?

During pregnancy, your cervix is sealed by a plug of "jelly-like" mucus that helps keep infections out. This plug comes out near the end of pregnancy and is accompanied by some blood. This may mean that labor is about to start; the bloody show may happen days or even weeks before the start of labor.

What does it mean when my "water breaks"?

The "water" is really the amniotic fluid that surrounds your baby. As your cervix dilates from the pressure of contractions, the sac surrounding your baby breaks, releasing the amniotic fluid. It may gush out or leak out slowly and is usually clear with little odor. If you think your water is leaking or it breaks, contact your doctor or midwife. If your water breaks and you're not in labor yet, you will most likely go into labor within 24 to 48 hours. If your water does not break on its own and it's time for your baby to be born, your doctor or midwife may break it.

What happens during each of the three stages of labor?

Begins with regular contractions, which cause your cervix to open (dilate), and ends when your cervix is fully open (about 10 cm in diameter). As your contractions become more intense, your cervix will soften, thin out, and open. You may be offered medication for pain relief at this time. Stage one of labor usually lasts eight to 14 hours. However this can vary. As the first stage of labor ends, you may enter into an intense stage of labor called "transition".

Begins when your cervix is fully open and ends with the birth of your baby. If your water hasn't broken on its own by now, your doctor or midwife may break it for you. If you are delivering vaginally, you will be asked to push during this stage. You may have a bowel movement; don't be embarrassed. This is involuntary and quite common while you are pushing. This stage can take as little as several minutes or as long as several hours. As a general rule, first babies take longer.

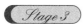

Begins after your baby is born and ends with the delivery of the afterbirth (placenta). This stage of labor can take a few minutes or last for an hour or more. You may need to push a bit to deliver the placenta. Breastfeeding your baby may help speed things up by stimulating the release of a hormone called oxytocin, which causes contractions. If you require stitching because of an episiotomy or natural tearing, this will be done soon after the placenta is delivered.

Why might labor be induced?

There are many reasons to "induce" or start labor.

Here Are Some Common Reasons to Induce Labor

You have carried your baby for 41 or 42 weeks and haven't gone into labor.

Your baby's growth has slowed down or stopped.

You develop preeclampsia.

You have placental insufficiency (when the placenta is not nourishing your baby properly).

You have a medical condition that requires an early delivery for the safety of you or your baby.

You are carrying multiple births. (Deliveries tend to come a few weeks earlier for each additional baby.)

What is preeclampsia?

Preeclampsia is a condition that develops in the mother during pregnancy. Symptoms can include high blood pressure; protein in the urine; weight gain from excessive fluid retention; headaches; nausea; vomiting; blurred vision; abdominal pain; and swelling in the ankles, legs, and fingers. Kidney and liver damage can occur if left untreated. Preeclampsia can be dangerous to both you and your baby. High blood pressure can reduce blood flow, depriving oxygen and nutrients to your baby. Severe preeclampsia means that your baby may need to be delivered early.

What is a cesarean birth and when might my doctor decide that I need one?

A cesarean birth is when your baby is lifted out of your womb through a cut in your abdomen. A planned cesarean birth may be scheduled when you've had a prior "c-section"; your baby is too large to deliver vaginally; your pelvis is too small; you are carrying multiple births; or you have a condition, such as AIDS, diabetes, or placenta previa (when the placenta or "afterbirth" covers the cervix). An emergency cesarean birth may be done if your blood pressure becomes dangerously high during labor, your baby is showing signs of distress, or if a problem occurs before or during labor that puts you or your baby in jeopardy.

What is an Apgar score?

An Apgar score is the result of a simple test used to measure how well a baby is doing in the first few minutes of life. It's done one minute after birth and then again five minutes after birth. A value from 0 to 2 to is given to each of the five signs; the numbers are then added together. An Apgar score of 7 or more (out of 10) indicates the baby is in good condition. A score between 4 and 6 may mean the baby is having a problem or needs help breathing. A score under 4 means he or she may need lifesaving techniques. Even if the score is low, the baby may recover quickly and be fine. The test is only used to tell which babies need closer short-term monitoring.

APGAR TEST

Sign	0 points	1 point	2 points	Score
Heart rate	Absent	Slow	>100/minute	
Breathing	Absent	Slow	Good; Crying	
Muscle tone	Limp	Some tone	Active motion	
Response to stimulus	None	Some Response	Sneezes/Coughs	
Color of body	Pale/Blue	Blue/Pink	Pink all over	

Total Apgar Score: ☞

JOURNAL
Babies

CONCEPTION AND

Pregnancy Journal

ABOUT YOUR CONCEPTION AND
Pregnancy Journal

Congratulations on your decision to use J O U R N A L *Babies*:
Your Personal Conception and Pregnancy Organizer. By keeping this journal,
you can plan, prepare, and preserve one of the most important events
in your life — childbirth. Planning, before and during pregnancy,
can help you achieve your goal of delivering a healthy baby.

If you are trying to get pregnant, use the monthly conception planner on pages 63 to
65 to track the fertile days in your menstrual cycle. This will help you determine the days you
are most likely to become pregnant. See the instructions on page 62 to learn how to use the
conception planner. If you need more conception planner pages, you may photocopy these pages.

If you are already pregnant, begin using this journal on page 76. As you prepare for your new
arrival, use the pages provided to record your:
- Questions and concerns for your health care provider.
- Hospital checklist.
- Weight throughout the pregnancy.
- Special memories.

Use the month-by-month pregnancy calendar pages to track doctor's appointments,
special tests and procedures, and each week of pregnancy. Instructions on
how to use the monthly calendar organizers are found on page 74.

Keep J O U R N A L *Babies* with you until delivery. It's the perfect planning tool
and on-going record of your conception, pregnancy, and delivery experience.

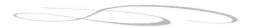

CONCEPTION PLANNER

Instructions

Begin using the Monthly Conception Planner on the
first day of your menstrual period. Cycle day 1 is the first day of your
menstrual period. Record this date above "cycle day 1" on the planner.

Each consecutive day, do the following:

- Record the date above the cycle day (see sample below).
- Place a checkmark (✓) in the appropriate box if you had
  intercourse (or insemination).
- Circle the cycle day when you receive a positive ovulation test result if you
  are using an ovulation predictor kit.
- Record your basal body temperature (BBT) in the space provided
  if you are monitoring your BBT.
- Use a new planner on the first day of your next menstrual period if you
  don't conceive. The sample planner is based on a 28-day menstrual cycle.

  Cycle day 1 (i.e., first day of period) was March 8th.

Monthly Conception Planner Sample

Date	3/8	3/9	3/10	3/11	3/12	3/13	3/14	3/15	3/16	3/17	3/18	3/19	3/20	3/21	3/22	3/23	3/24	3/25	3/26	3/27
Cycle Day	1	2	3	4	5	6	7	8	9	10	11	12	(13)	14	15	16	17	18	19	20
Intercourse									✓		✓		✓	✓	✓					✓
BBT	97.2	97.4	97.3	97.4	97.4	97.4	97.6	97.4	97.4	97.5	97.3	97.4	97.4	97	98	98	98.2	98	98	98.2

Date	3/28	3/29	3/30	3/31	4/1	4/2	4/3	4/4												
Cycle Day	21	22	23	24	25	26	27	28	29	30	31	32	33	34	35	36	37	38	39	40
Intercourse		✓				✓														
BBT	98.2	98	98	98.2	98.2	98	98	97.4												

Monthly Conception Planner

Date																				
Cycle Day	1	2	3	4	5	6	7	8	9	10	11	12	13	14	15	16	17	18	19	20
Intercourse																				
BBT																				
Date																				
Cycle Day	21	22	23	24	25	26	27	28	29	30	31	32	33	34	35	36	37	38	39	40
Intercourse																				
BBT																				

Monthly Conception Planner

Date																				
Cycle Day	1	2	3	4	5	6	7	8	9	10	11	12	13	14	15	16	17	18	19	20
Intercourse																				
BBT																				
Date																				
Cycle Day	21	22	23	24	25	26	27	28	29	30	31	32	33	34	35	36	37	38	39	40
Intercourse																				
BBT																				

Monthly Conception Planner

Date																				
Cycle Day	1	2	3	4	5	6	7	8	9	10	11	12	13	14	15	16	17	18	19	20
Intercourse																				
BBT																				
Date																				
Cycle Day	21	22	23	24	25	26	27	28	29	30	31	32	33	34	35	36	37	38	39	40
Intercourse																				
BBT																				

Monthly Conception Planner

Date																				
Cycle Day	1	2	3	4	5	6	7	8	9	10	11	12	13	14	15	16	17	18	19	20
Intercourse																				
BBT																				
Date																				
Cycle Day	21	22	23	24	25	26	27	28	29	30	31	32	33	34	35	36	37	38	39	40
Intercourse																				
BBT																				

Monthly Conception Planner

Date																				
Cycle Day	1	2	3	4	5	6	7	8	9	10	11	12	13	14	15	16	17	18	19	20
Intercourse																				
BBT																				
Date																				
Cycle Day	21	22	23	24	25	26	27	28	29	30	31	32	33	34	35	36	37	38	39	40
Intercourse																				
BBT																				

Monthly Conception Planner

Date																				
Cycle Day	1	2	3	4	5	6	7	8	9	10	11	12	13	14	15	16	17	18	19	20
Intercourse																				
BBT																				
Date																				
Cycle Day	21	22	23	24	25	26	27	28	29	30	31	32	33	34	35	36	37	38	39	40
Intercourse																				
BBT																				

A R E Y O U P R E G N A N T Y E T ?

Use the chart below to record the results of your pregnancy test(s).

Date	Type of Test	Result	Comments and Thoughts
/ /	☐ Urine ☐ Blood	☐ Positive ☐ Negative	
/ /	☐ Urine ☐ Blood	☐ Positive ☐ Negative	
/ /	☐ Urine ☐ Blood	☐ Positive ☐ Negative	
/ /	☐ Urine ☐ Blood	☐ Positive ☐ Negative	
/ /	☐ Urine ☐ Blood	☐ Positive ☐ Negative	
/ /	☐ Urine ☐ Blood	☐ Positive ☐ Negative	
/ /	☐ Urine ☐ Blood	☐ Positive ☐ Negative	
/ /	☐ Urine ☐ Blood	☐ Positive ☐ Negative	
/ /	☐ Urine ☐ Blood	☐ Positive ☐ Negative	
/ /	☐ Urine ☐ Blood	☐ Positive ☐ Negative	

FIRST SIGNS OF PREGNANCY

Congratulations!

Date	Sign of Pregnancy	Comments and Thoughts
/ /		
/ /		
/ /		
/ /		
/ /		

Start date of last menstrual period __/ /__   Date menstrual period was due __/ /__

FAVORITE NAMES FOR BABY

Boy's Names

Girl's Names

Daily Nutrition Quick-Check

Give your baby the best possible start by eating well during your pregnancy. Remember — when you eat healthy — so does your developing baby. Use the checklist below as a guideline to help you choose a variety of nutritious foods each day.

Daily Nutrition Checklist	Sample Foods & Serving Sizes *One serving is equal to any of the following items:*
☑ *I eat 8 or more servings of grains*	1/2 small bagel or English muffin 1 slice whole grain bread 1/2 cup cooked rice, pasta, or cereal 1 ounce ready-to-eat cereal 1 (6-inch) tortilla
☑ *I eat 4 or more servings of fruit*	1 medium-sized fresh fruit 1/2 cup frozen, cooked, or canned fruit 1/4 cup dried fruit 3/4 cup fruit juice
☑ *I eat 4 or more servings of vegetables*	1/2 cup cooked vegetables 1 cup raw leafy vegetables 3/4 cup vegetable juice
☑ *I eat 4 or more servings of calcium-rich foods*	1 cup milk or yogurt 1 cup calcium-fortified orange juice or soy beverage 1 1/2 ounces natural cheese 2 ounces processed cheese
☑ *I eat 3 servings of protein foods.*	2 to 3 ounces lean meat, fish, or poultry 2 eggs or 1/2 cup egg substitute 1/2 cup tuna, tofu, or legumes 2 tablespoons peanut butter 1/4 cup nuts
☑ *I limit fatty foods and sweets*	Fried foods, full-fat dairy products, regular sodas, desserts, and fast foods.
☑ *I drink 8 to 10 glasses of water/fluid.*	1 cup plain or sparkling water 1 cup decaffeinated coffee or tea Other beverages, such as milk and juice, also count as fluid.
☑ *I eat a variety of iron-rich foods.*	Iron-fortified cereals, eggs, beef, chicken, prune juice, soybeans, tofu, legumes, lentils, and quinoa.
☑ *I eat a variety of vitamin C-rich foods.*	Citrus fruits, berries, kiwifruit, mangoes, papayas, leafy green vegetables, tomatoes, cauliflower, bell peppers, and cabbage.
☑ *I eat a variety of fiber-rich foods.*	Whole grain breads, fiber-rich cereals, wheat germ, wheat bran, fruits, vegetables, nuts, seeds, and legumes.
☑ *I take my prenatal vitamin as prescribed by my physician.*	Talk to your physician about the amount of folic acid that's right for you. Current recommendations are at least 400 micrograms.

Find out how your eating habits stack up against the *Eating Expectantly Food Guide Pyramid*, (page 44), by keeping a food log. Record everything you eat and drink for four days. Place a checkmark (X) in the food group box (below) for each food eaten. Assess your physical activity level by placing a checkmark (X) in one box for every 10 minutes of activity. Eating well and staying active is an important part of a healthy pregnancy.

Time	Foods and Beverages	Amount
7:00	Cereal	1 1/2 cups
	Skim Milk	1 cup
	Banana	1 medium
10:00	Bagel with P.B + jelly	1/2 w 1-Tbsp. P.B
	Orange juice	1 cup
	Mineral water	20oz bottle
12:15	Sandwich–2 slices of bread	2 slices
	Mayo /lettuce	1 Tbsp.
	Cheese / shaved turkey	1 slice; 2 ounces
	Baby Carrots –raw	about 8
	Pudding cup	1/2 cup
	Apple	1 medium
	Mineral water	10oz (1/2 bottle)
3:00	Strawberry– flavor yogurt	6 oz
	Whole Wheat crackers	about 8
	Mineral Water	10oz (1/2 bottle)
6:15	Beef Stirfry	1 1/2 cups TOTAL
	(Round steak, mushrooms, onions, broccoli,	
	peapods, carrots, celery)	
	Rice	3/4 cup
	Melon cubes	1 cup
	Skim Milk	1 cup
8:45	Popcorn / mineral water/ Frozen yogurt bar	6 cups / 10oz / 1 bar

GRAINS 8 OR MORE SERVINGS — X X X X / X X X X X

FRUIT 4 OR MORE SERVINGS — X X X / X X ☐

VEGETABLE 4 OR MORE SERVINGS — X X X / X X ☐

DAIRY 4 OR MORE SERVINGS — X X ☐ / X X ☐

PROTEIN 3 OR MORE SERVINGS — X X X ☐ ☐

FAT SPARINGLY — X X X X ☐

SWEETS SPARINGLY — X X ☐

WATER / FLUID 8 TO 10 CUPS — X X X X / X X X ☐

PHYICAL ACTIVITY — X X X ☐ ☐ / X X ☐ ☐

Goals and comments:

1.) Eat Breakfast   2) Take short walks at breaktime

3.) Fill my glass at the drink fountain to have water at my desk.

DAILY FOOD LOG

DATE
/ /

Time	Foods and Beverages	Amount

GRAINS
8 OR MORE SERVINGS

FRUIT
4 OR MORE SERVINGS

VEGETABLE
4 OR MORE SERVINGS

DAIRY
4 OR MORE SERVINGS

PROTEIN
3 OR MORE SERVINGS

FAT
SPARINGLY

SWEETS
SPARINGLY

WATER / FLUID
8 TO 10 CUPS

PHYICAL ACTIVITY
| 10 MIN | 10 MIN | 10 MIN | 10 MIN |
| 10 MIN | 10 MIN | 10 MIN | 10 MIN |

Goals and comments:

Daily Food Log

Time	Foods and Beverages	Amount

GRAINS
8 OR MORE SERVINGS

FRUIT
4 OR MORE SERVINGS

VEGETABLE
4 OR MORE SERVINGS

DAIRY
4 OR MORE SERVINGS

PROTEIN
3 OR MORE SERVINGS

FAT
SPARINGLY

SWEETS
SPARINGLY

WATER / FLUID
8 TO 10 CUPS

PHYICAL ACTIVITY
10 MIN / 10 MIN / 10 MIN / 10 MIN
10 MIN / 10 MIN / 10 MIN / 10 MIN

Goals and comments:

Daily Food Log

Time	Foods and Beverages	Amount

GRAINS
8 OR MORE SERVINGS
☐ ☐ ☐ ☐ ☐
☐ ☐ ☐ ☐ ☐

FRUIT
4 OR MORE SERVINGS
☐ ☐ ☐
☐ ☐ ☐

VEGETABLE
4 OR MORE SERVINGS
☐ ☐ ☐
☐ ☐ ☐

DAIRY
4 OR MORE SERVINGS
☐ ☐ ☐
☐ ☐ ☐

PROTEIN
3 OR MORE SERVINGS
☐ ☐ ☐ ☐ ☐

FAT
SPARINGLY
☐ ☐ ☐ ☐ ☐

SWEETS
SPARINGLY
☐ ☐ ☐

WATER / FLUID
8 TO 10 CUPS
☐ ☐ ☐ ☐ ☐
☐ ☐ ☐ ☐ ☐

Goals and comments:

PHYICAL ACTIVITY
| 10 MIN | 10 MIN | 10 MIN | 10 MIN |
| 10 MIN | 10 MIN | 10 MIN | 10 MIN |

DAILY FOOD LOG

DATE ___/___/___

Time	Foods and Beverages	Amount

GRAINS
8 OR MORE SERVINGS
☐☐☐☐☐
☐☐☐☐☐

FRUIT
4 OR MORE SERVINGS
☐☐☐
☐

VEGETABLE
4 OR MORE SERVINGS
☐☐☐
☐☐☐

DAIRY
4 OR MORE SERVINGS
☐☐☐
☐☐☐

PROTEIN
3 OR MORE SERVINGS
☐☐☐☐☐

FAT
SPARINGLY
☐☐☐☐☐

SWEETS
SPARINGLY
☐☐☐

WATER / FLUID
8 TO 10 CUPS
☐☐☐☐☐
☐☐☐☐☐

PHYICAL ACTIVITY
| 10 MIN | 10 MIN | 10 MIN | 10 MIN |
| 10 MIN | 10 MIN | 10 MIN | 10 MIN |

Goals and comments:

_____

_____

PREGNANCY CALENDAR

Instructions

Use the month-by-month pregnancy calendars
on the following pages:

If you know how many weeks pregnant you are, go to the correct week
of pregnancy. Then, take a calendar for the current year and write the dates in
the boxes (upper right corner) for each day for the remaining weeks of pregnancy.

If you don't know how many weeks pregnant you are, first determine
the date and day of the week of the **first day of your last menstrual period (LMP).**
Write this date in the correct box in "Week 1" on page 77. Then, take a calendar
for the current year and write in the dates in the boxes (upper right corner) for the
remaining weeks of pregnancy.

On the next page is a sample calendar based on a woman who started her last
menstrual period on Wednesday, March 8.

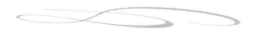

Sample Calendar

March–April
Month / Year

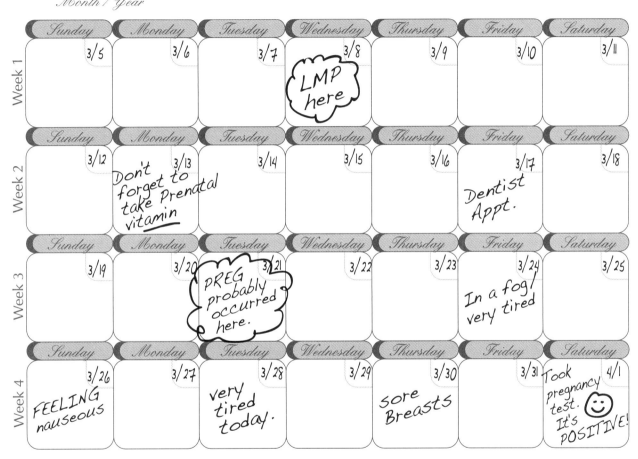

Week 1

Sunday	Monday	Tuesday	Wednesday	Thursday	Friday	Saturday
3/5	3/6	3/7	3/8 LMP here	3/9	3/10	3/11

Week 2

Sunday	Monday	Tuesday	Wednesday	Thursday	Friday	Saturday
3/12	3/13 Don't forget to take Prenatal vitamin	3/14	3/15	3/16	3/17 Dentist Appt.	3/18

Week 3

Sunday	Monday	Tuesday	Wednesday	Thursday	Friday	Saturday
3/19	3/20	3/21 PREG probably occurred here.	3/22	3/23	3/24 In a fog/ very tired	3/25

Week 4

Sunday	Monday	Tuesday	Wednesday	Thursday	Friday	Saturday
3/26 FEELING nauseous	3/27	3/28 very tired today.	3/29	3/30 sore Breasts	3/31	4/1 Took pregnancy test. ☺ It's POSITIVE!

(Note: The first day of your last menstrual period (LMP) marks the beginning of your pregnancy, according to the medical profession. By the time conception takes place, you are considered to be two weeks pregnant.)

THE FIRST
Month of Pregnancy

Baby's Development: The moment of conception has occurred, and you now have a unique individual growing inside of your womb. After just one week, the small cluster of cells attaches itself to the wall of your uterus and continues to divide. This is known as "implantation".

Mom's Changes: By the end of the month, you may already feel pregnant. Early signs of pregnancy may include enlarged and/or tender breasts, nausea, fatigue, frequent urination, and constipation. Also, certain tastes and smells may be enhanced.

Questions for your health care provider:

Date	Questions	Answers

Memories and thoughts:

Month / Year

	Sunday	Monday	Tuesday	Wednesday	Thursday	Friday	Saturday
Week 1							
	First trimester begins.			Record the date of the first day of your LMP here in week 1.			
Week 2	Sunday	Monday	Tuesday	Wednesday	Thursday	Friday	Saturday
Week 3	Sunday	Monday	Tuesday	Wednesday	Thursday	Friday	Saturday
Week 4	Sunday	Monday	Tuesday	Wednesday	Thursday	Friday	Saturday

Baby's Size: Smaller than this dot ⟶ 👉

THE SECOND
Month of Pregnancy

Baby's Development: Your baby's heart begins to beat, and blood begins to flow. The eyes, upper lip, teeth, arms, fingers, ears, legs, lungs, stomach, nervous system, spinal cord, brain, and internal organs start to develop. Your baby looks more like a tadpole than a person.

Mom's Changes: You may be feeling very emotional and/or nauseous throughout the day and/or night. This is common while your body adjusts to pregnancy. Your uterus is now the size of a tennis ball.

Questions for your health care provider:

Date	Questions	Answers

Memories and thoughts:

_____

_____

_____

_____

_____

_____

Month / Year

	Sunday	Monday	Tuesday	Wednesday	Thursday	Friday	Saturday
Week 5							
Week 6	Sunday	Monday	Tuesday	Wednesday	Thursday	Friday	Saturday
Week 7	Sunday	Monday	Tuesday	Wednesday	Thursday	Friday	Saturday
Week 8	Sunday	Monday	Tuesday	Wednesday	Thursday	Friday	Saturday

Baby's Length (crown to rump): ~ $1/2$ inch, Weight: ~ .06 ounces

THE THIRD
Month of Pregnancy

Baby's Development: Your baby's toes, genitals, neck, and fingernails are forming. All of the major organs are now fully formed, and urine is produced. The arms and legs are beginning to move, and the heart is pumping blood to all parts of your baby's body.

Mom's Changes: Your uterus has begun to enlarge, pressing on your bladder so that you may need to urinate more often. Your metabolism increases, which may cause you to feel hot or flushed. As your lung capacity increases, you may feel as if you are breathing more quickly.

Questions for your health care provider:

Date	Questions	Answers

Memories and thoughts:

_____

_____

_____

_____

_____

_____

Month / Year

	Sunday	Monday	Tuesday	Wednesday	Thursday	Friday	Saturday
Week 9							
Week 10							
Week 11							
Week 12	First Trimester Ends						

Baby's Length (crown to rump): ~ 2 1/2 inches, Weight: ~ 1/2 ounce

THE FOURTH
Month of Pregnancy

Baby's Development: Congratulations! You've now completed your first trimester. In the second trimester, your baby will start to grow more rapidly — about two inches per month. Your baby is starting to resemble a tiny person, although its head still makes up more than one-third of its length.

Mom's Changes: You may be feeling better. Morning sickness is usually gone by now. Your appetite and energy return, and you may urinate less often. Your breasts continue to swell, dark veins appear, and the skin around your nipples (areola) darkens. Your uterus is about the size of a grapefruit.

Questions for your health care provider:

Date	Questions	Answers

Memories and thoughts:

_____

_____

_____

_____

_____

_____

Month / Year

	Sunday	Monday	Tuesday	Wednesday	Thursday	Friday	Saturday
Week 13							
	Second Trimester Begins						
Week 14							
Week 15							
Week 16							

Baby's Length (crown to rump): ~ 4 3/4 inches, Weight: ~ 4 1/2 ounces

THE FIFTH
Month of Pregnancy

Baby's Development: Your baby develops a layer of fat beneath the skin, and soft hair (lanugo) covers the skin. Your baby can hear and may respond to noises. Although the eyes are shut, they can move from side to side. Muscle strength increases, allowing for more coordinated movements.

Mom's Changes: You may be able to feel your baby fluttering around in your body. You also may feel small false contractions known as "Braxton-Hicks' contractions". Your breasts may secrete a milky substance, and a dark line down the center of your stomach (linea nigra) may be noticeable.

Questions for your health care provider:

Date	Questions	Answers

Memories and thoughts:

_____

_____

_____

_____

_____

_____

_____

Month / Year

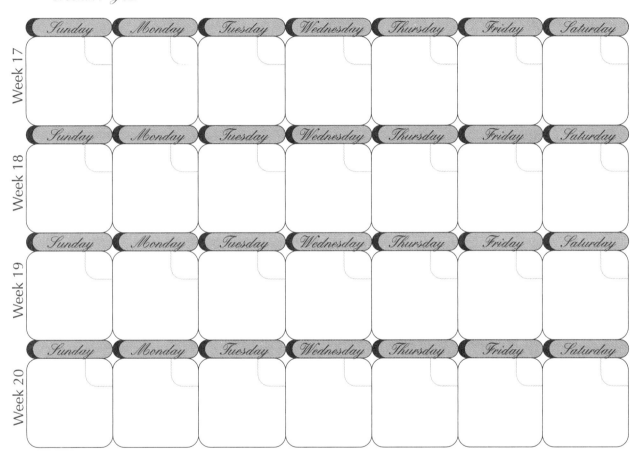

	Sunday	Monday	Tuesday	Wednesday	Thursday	Friday	Saturday
Week 17							
Week 18							
Week 19							
Week 20							

BABY'S Length (crown to rump): ~ 6 1/3 inches, Weight: ~ 12 ounces

THE SIXTH
Month of Pregnancy

Baby's Development: All of your baby's major organs are functioning, with the exception of the lungs. He or she can now suck its thumb, smile, frown, open and close its mouth and eyes, cough, hiccup, and tumble around in your womb as strength and dexterity increase.

Mom's Changes: Your heart is working harder because of increased blood volume. Since your uterus is pressing on major blood vessels, you may feel faint when you lie on your back, or when you stand for a while. Your gums may become sensitive, and your moles and freckles may darken.

Questions for your health care provider:

Date	Questions	Answers

Memories and thoughts:

_____

_____

_____

_____

_____

_____

_____

Month / Year

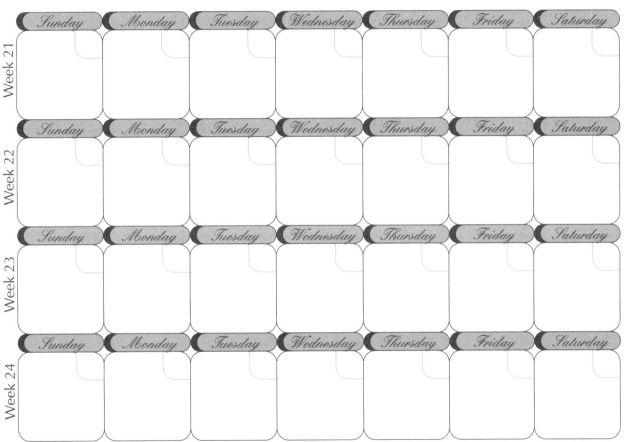

	Sunday	Monday	Tuesday	Wednesday	Thursday	Friday	Saturday
Week 21							
Week 22							
Week 23							
Week 24							

BABY'S Length (crown to rump): ~ 8 inches, Weight: ~ 1 1/2 pounds

THE SEVENTH
Month of Pregnancy

Baby's Development: Your baby's head is more proportionate with the rest of its body, and it may be covered with hair. Eyebrows and eyelashes appear. A white, thick protective waxy coating known as "vernix" covers the skin and acts as an insulator.

Mom's Changes: You may see your stomach move as your baby moves, and others may be able to feel these movements with their hands. By now, your baby is moving around quite vigorously, often kicking and punching, and perhaps interrupting your sleep and/or conversations.

Questions for your health care provider:

Date	Questions	Answers

Memories and thoughts:

_____

_____

_____

_____

_____

_____

Month / Year

	Sunday	Monday	Tuesday	Wednesday	Thursday	Friday	Saturday
Week 25							
Week 26							
Week 27							
Week 28							

Second Trimester Ends

Third Trimester Begins

Baby's Length (crown to rump): ~ 10 inches, Weight: ~ 2 1/2 pounds

THE EIGHTH
Month of Pregnancy

Baby's Development: The substance "surfactant", which aids in breathing, is now present in the lungs and greatly increases your baby's chance of survival. Your baby may be in a "heads-down" position, pressing on your bladder — so again, you may need to urinate more often.

Mom's Changes: You may experience strong Braxton-Hicks[1] contractions, heartburn, shortness of breath, leg cramps, and/or swelling in your feet and legs. As your supporting ligaments soften (so that your pelvis can expand in preparation for delivery), you may have some lower back pain.

Questions for your health care provider:

Date	Questions	Answers

Memories and thoughts:

_____

_____

_____

_____

_____

_____

Month / Year

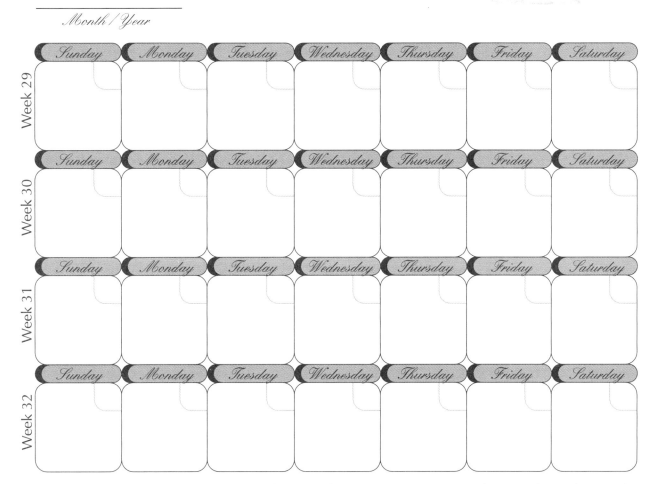

	Sunday	Monday	Tuesday	Wednesday	Thursday	Friday	Saturday
Week 29							
Week 30							
Week 31							
Week 32							

Baby's Length (crown to rump): ~ 12 inches, Weight: ~ 3 1/2 pounds

THE NINTH
Month of Pregnancy

Baby's Development: Although your baby still needs to put on more weight for insulation, its head is now in proportion with the rest of its body, and he or she looks like a tiny person. When its head drops into your pelvis — this is called "lightening".

Mom's Changes: You may feel the need to "nest" or clean — in order to get things ready for your new arrival. You may feel tired, forgetful, seem clumsy, and/or have difficulty sleeping. The pressure on your stomach and lungs decreases, reducing symptoms of heartburn and shortness of breath.

Questions for your health care provider:

Date	Questions	Answers

Memories and thoughts:

Month / Year

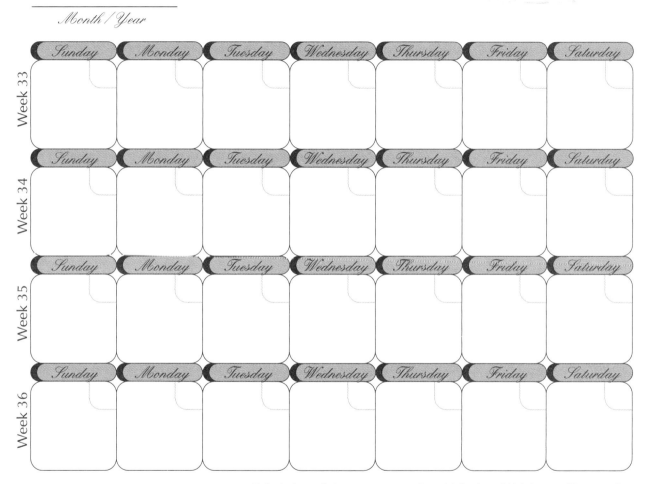

	Sunday	Monday	Tuesday	Wednesday	Thursday	Friday	Saturday
Week 33							
Week 34							
Week 35							
Week 36							

Baby's Length (crown to rump): ~ 13 inches, Weight: ~ 5 1/2 pounds

THE TENTH
Month of Pregnancy

Baby's Development: Your baby is gaining weight at the rate of one ounce each day or about one-half pound each week. Its skin is soft and smooth, the lanugo has almost disappeared, and the lungs are fully formed. Its eyes will be blue at birth, and will open when he or she is awake.

Mom's Changes: You're probably anxious to meet your baby. You may have more noticeable contractions (pre-labor). When labor begins, you may see a "mucus plug" with a little blood, as your cervix starts to open. If your water breaks or true labor begins — call your health care provider. It's time!

Questions for your health care provider:

Date	Questions	Answers

Memories and thoughts:

_____

_____

_____

_____

_____

_____

Month / Year

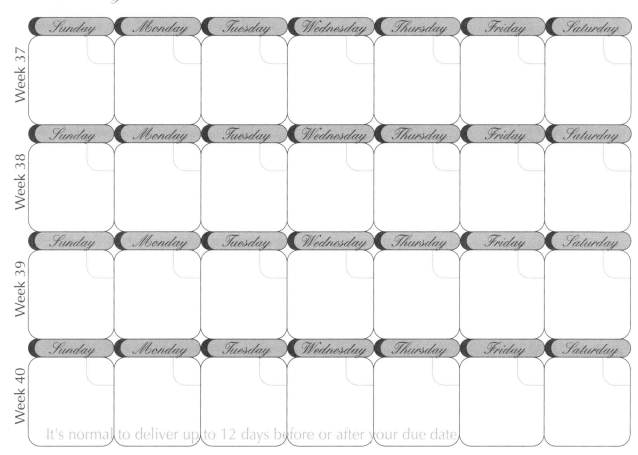

	Sunday	Monday	Tuesday	Wednesday	Thursday	Friday	Saturday
Week 37							
Week 38							
Week 39							
Week 40							

It's normal to deliver up to 12 days before or after your due date.

Baby reaches his or her birth length and weight.

Childbirth Education

Classes Attended

Date	Class	Things to Remember
/ /		
/ /		
/ /		
/ /		
/ /		
/ /		
/ /		
/ /		
/ /		
/ /		

HOSPITAL CHECKLIST

For You

- ☐ Books/magazines
- ☐ Breast pads/nursing bra
- ☐ Camera/camcorder/film
- ☐ Change/money
- ☐ Comb/hair brush
- ☐ Conditioner/shampoo
- ☐ Cosmetics
- ☐ Curling iron/hair dryer
- ☐ Deodorant/lotion/soap
- ☐ Insurance card
- ☐ Journal Babies/pen
- ☐ Lip balm
- ☐ Loose-fitting outfit
- ☐ Nursing nightgown/pajamas
- ☐ Pillow
- ☐ Razor
- ☐ Robe
- ☐ Slippers/socks
- ☐ Snacks
- ☐ Sweater
- ☐ Tennis ball (for use during back labor)
- ☐ Toothbrush/toothpaste
- ☐ Underwear
- ☐ Watch with second hand

For Baby

- ☐ Baby book
- ☐ Baby nail scissors or clippers
- ☐ Bag (to bring things home)
- ☐ Blanket
- ☐ Booties
- ☐ Car seat
- ☐ Coat/sweater
- ☐ Comb/hair brush
- ☐ Diapers (usually provided)
- ☐ Hat
- ☐ Outfit/sleeper
- ☐ Pacifier

Other _____   _____
_____   _____
_____   _____
_____   _____

MOM'S TEST RESULTS

(e.g., AFP, amniocentesis, glucose tolerance test, ultrasound)

Date	Type of Test	Results
__/__/__		
__/__/__		
__/__/__		
__/__/__		
__/__/__		

PEOPLE TO CALL WHEN BABY ARRIVES

Name	Telephone Number(s)

CHILDBIRTH PLAN

I will deliver my baby: ☐ at home   ☐ in a hospital   ☐ in a birthing center

Name and telephone number of doctor or midwife:_____

Name, address, and telephone number of hospital or birthing center: _____
_____

Name and telephone number of person who will drive me to the hospital:_____

Name and telephone number of my childbirth partner and coach: _____

Names of siblings, friends, or relatives attending the birth:_____
_____

I would like to be offered medication for pain relief: ☐ yes   ☐ no   If yes, type: _____

Name of person to cut the umbilical cord:_____

I would like to have my baby placed directly on my abdomen after delivery if possible: ☐ yes   ☐ no

My feelings on having an episiotomy are:_____

I would like to bring a camera or camcorder in the delivery room: ☐ yes   ☐ no

I would like to watch my baby being born: ☐ yes   ☐ no

I would like my baby to stay in the room with me (birth in) if possible: ☐ yes   ☐ no

I plan to: ☐ breastfeed   ☐ bottle feed   ☐ combination of both

If I have a boy, will I/we have him circumcised?   ☐ yes   ☐ no

Other Thoughts:
_____
_____

CHILDBIRTH DIARY

Use the space below to record your labor and delivery experience.

Memories and thoughts:

PREGNANCY WEIGHT RECORD

Step 1:
Record your pre-pregnancy weight and your recommended weight gain in the boxes.

Step 2:
Place your current weight in the "Weight" column, next to the appropriate "Week" of pregnancy (on the weeks when you do weigh-in).

Step 3:
Calculate the total number of pounds you've gained (or lost) by **subtracting your pre-pregnancy weight from your current weight;** record this number in the "total" column. Repeat this calculation each time you weigh-in to keep a running total of your pregnancy weight gain.

Pre-pregnancy Weight ( )   Recommended Weight Gain ( )

First Trimester			Second Trimester			Third Trimester		
Week	Weight	Total	Week	Weight	Total	Week	Weight	Total
1			13			26		
2			14			27		
3			15			28		
4			16			29		
5			17			30		
6			18			31		
7			19			32		
8			20			33		
9			21			34		
10			22			35		
11			23			36		
12			24			37		
			25			38		
						39		
						40		

Total Weight Gain—

LOOK WHO'S HERE!

Baby's Name *first* _____ *middle* _____ *last* _____

Date of Birth _____ **Day of Week** _____

Time of Birth _____ **Place of Birth** _____

Baby's Weight _____ **Baby's Length** _____

Other _____ **Other** _____

BABY'S TEST RESULTS

(e.g., Apgar, Brazelton, PKU)

Date	Type of Test	Results
/ /		
/ /		
/ /		
/ /		
/ /		

REFERENCES

Fulghum, Bruce and Debra; and Thatcher, Samuel. *Making a Baby: Everything You Need to Know to Get Pregnant.* New York: The Ballantine Publishing Group, 2000.

Reynolds, Karina; Lees, Christoph; and McCartan, Grainne. *Pregnancy and Birth: Your Questions Answered.* New York: DK Publishing, Inc., 1997.

Seibel, Machelle M. *Infertility: A Comprehensive Text. 2nd ed.* Connecticut: Appleton & Lange Press, 1997.

Swinney, Bridget; and Anderson, Tracey. *Eating Expectantly: A Practical and Tasty Guide to Prenatal Nutrition.* Minnesota: Meadowbrook Press, 2000.

The American College of Obstetricians and Gynecologists (ACOG). *Planning for Pregnancy, Birth and Beyond. 2nd ed.* Washington, DC: ACOG, 1995.

Tan, S.L.; Jacobs, Howard S., and Seibel, Machelle M. *Infertility: Your Questions Answered.* New York: Birch Lane Press, Carol Publishing Group, 1995.

PASSAGES

IT IS DARK. DARK AND DESERTED. I AM ALONE.
NOT SPEAKING, BARELY MOVING, FLOATING THROUGH LIFE.

NOTHING COULD HAVE PREPARED ME FOR WHAT HAPPENED,
OR FOR WHAT WAS TO COME.
NOT THE MONTHS OF INTIMACY, OF GROWING TOGETHER,
OF BEING ENVELOPED IN LOVE.

ONE DAY, ALMOST WITHOUT WARNING,
THE PRESSURE BEGAN TO BUILD.
SLOWLY AT FIRST, THEN SLOWLY GREATER,
UNTIL THE FORCE OF IT LEFT ME
POUNDING MY HEAD AGAINST THE WALL—
AGAIN AND AGAIN!

THE STRAIN WAS OVERWHELMING. I LONGED
TO RELIEVE THE TENSION IN MY BODY.
I FELT A RUPTURE.

ARCHING MY NECK, SCRUNCHING MY FACE,
PEERING HEAVENLY FOR LIGHT AND FOR AIR
I GASPED, THEN I CRIED.

AND SUDDENLY, I WAS BORN.

--Machelle M. Seibel

THE INDEX

ORDER FORM

HealthCheques™: JOURNAL *Babies*:
Your Personal Conception & Pregnancy Organizer

By Machelle Seibel, MD and Jane Stephenson, RD, CDE. Copyright 2002. This book is written for every woman who is planning on becoming pregnant or who is already pregnant. This book empowers women with an understanding of the pregnancy process from conception to delivery. It can maximize chances of conception by helping women pinpoint the fertile days in their menstrual cycle and answers questions about fertility, conception, assisted conception, pregnancy, and childbirth. The month-by-month pregnancy calendar pages help women record and organize the details of the pregnancy experience such as keeping track of doctor's appointments, special tests, and procedures.

_____ One JOURNAL *Babies* at $12.95

_____ **Special Value!** Two books or more for $11.00/each

_____ Shipping & Handling: Please add $3.00 for 1st book and $1.00 for each additional book.

_____ Total Enclosed   Circle Method of Payment: Check VISA MasterCard

Card Number _____ Expiration Date _____

Send to:
Name _____

Address _____

City _____ State _____ Zipcode _____

Mail to: APPLETREE PRESS, INC
151 Good Counsel Drive • Suite #125
Mankato, MN 56001

Toll-free 1-800-322-5679 • Fax (507) 345-3002
Website: www.appletree-press.com

ORDER FORM

HealthCheques™: JOURNAL *Babies*:
Your Personal Conception & Pregnancy Organizer

By Machelle Seibel, MD and Jane Stephenson, RD, CDE. Copyright 2002. This book is written for every woman who is planning on becoming pregnant or who is already pregnant. This book empowers women with an understanding of the pregnancy process from conception to delivery. It can maximize chances of conception by helping women pinpoint the fertile days in their menstrual cycle and answers questions about fertility, conception, assisted conception, pregnancy, and childbirth. The month-by-month pregnancy calendar pages help women record and organize the details of the pregnancy experience such as keeping track of doctor's appointments, special tests, and procedures.

_____ One JOURNAL *Babies* at $12.95

_____ **Special Value!** Two books or more for $11.00/each

_____ Shipping & Handling: Please add $3.00 for 1st book and $1.00 for each additional book.

_____ Total Enclosed   Circle Method of Payment: Check   VISA   MasterCard

Card Number _____ Expiration Date _____

Send to:
Name _____

Address _____

City _____ State _____ Zipcode _____

Mail to: APPLETREE PRESS, INC
151 Good Counsel Drive • Suite #125
Mankato, MN 56001

Toll-free 1-800-322-5679 • Fax (507) 345-3002
Website: www.appletree-press.com

ORDER FORM

HealthCheques™: JOURNAL *Babies*:
Your Personal Conception & Pregnancy Organizer

By Machelle Seibel, MD and Jane Stephenson, RD, CDE. Copyright 2002. This book is written for every woman who is planning on becoming pregnant or who is already pregnant. This book empowers women with an understanding of the pregnancy process from conception to delivery. It can maximize chances of conception by helping women pinpoint the fertile days in their menstrual cycle and answers questions about fertility, conception, assisted conception, pregnancy, and childbirth. The month-by-month pregnancy calendar pages help women record and organize the details of the pregnancy experience such as keeping track of doctor's appointments, special tests, and procedures.

_____ One JOURNAL *Babies* at $12.95

_____ **Special Value!** Two books or more for $11.00/each

_____ Shipping & Handling: Please add $3.00 for 1st book and $1.00 for each additional book.

_____ Total Enclosed   Circle Method of Payment: Check VISA MasterCard

Card Number _____ Expiration Date _____

Send to:
Name _____

Address _____

City _____ State _____ Zipcode _____

Mail to: APPLETREE PRESS, INC
151 Good Counsel Drive • Suite #125
Mankato, MN 56001

Toll-free 1-800-322-5679 • Fax (507) 345-3002
Website: www.appletree-press.com